DIABETES WON'T STOP ME

SHORT SUCCESS STORY ABOUT A PERSON WITH DIABETES

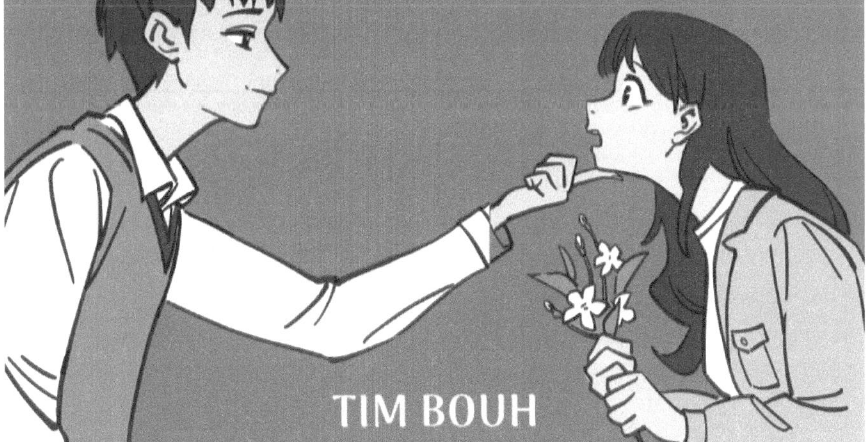

TIM BOUH

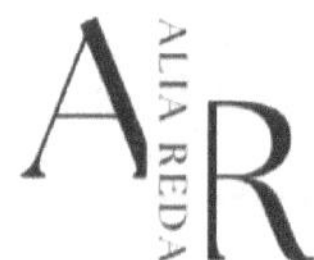

ALIAREDA © 2023

Introduction

Diabetes is a chronic condition that affects millions of people worldwide. The challenges that come with it can be overwhelming, but the stories of those who have overcome them are truly inspiring. In this book, we delve into the accounts of individuals who have successfully managed their diabetes and achieved their goals despite the odds.

These short success stories serve as a reminder that living with diabetes is not an insurmountable challenge, and that it is possible to lead a happy and fulfilling life with this condition. Whether you or someone you know is living with diabetes, these uplifting stories are sure to motivate and inspire you to take control of your health and achieve your dreams.

Book Outline

Short Success Story 21: Ashley

In addition to starting a support group in her community, Ashley has also been sharing her story and experiences on social media platforms. She believes that her journey can inspire others to take control of their diabetes and improve their health outcomes.

Ashley has also become an advocate for diabetes research and fundraising efforts. She participates in charity events and organizes local fundraising campaigns to support research on diabetes. She has made it her goal to spread awareness about the importance of diabetes management and to provide resources for individuals who are struggling with the disease.

Through her dedication and hard work, Ashley has achieved great success in her diabetes management journey. She continues to inspire and motivate others to take charge of their health and live their best lives, regardless of their health conditions.

Ashley's efforts have not gone unnoticed, and she has been recognized by numerous organizations for her contributions to diabetes education and advocacy. She has been invited to speak at conferences and events, both locally and nationally, where she shares her story and encourages others to take action.

Additionally, Ashley has started a non-profit organization focused on helping individuals with diabetes. The organization provides resources, education, and support for those with the disease, and also raises funds for diabetes research.

With the help of her support group, social media platform, and non-profit organization, Ashley has created a community of people who share similar experiences and challenges related to diabetes. She has built a network of individuals who inspire and support one another, and who are motivated to work together to improve their health outcomes and find a cure for diabetes.

Ashley's success story serves as an inspiration to others to never give up and to always keep fighting, even in the face of a chronic illness. Her determination, passion, and advocacy work have made a significant impact on the diabetes community and will continue to do so for years to come.

By educating and empowering others to manage their diabetes, Ashley has not only improved her own health outcomes but has also helped others do the same. Through her non-profit organization, Ashley has also contributed to diabetes research, which has the potential to lead to new treatment options and a potential cure. Her efforts have not only transformed her own life but also impacted the lives of countless others.

Ashley's story highlights the power of individual action and the impact it can have on a larger community. By sharing her personal experiences and advocating for diabetes management and research, she has created a movement that is making a difference in the lives of those with diabetes. Ashley is a shining example of how one person can make a significant impact in the world, and her legacy will continue to inspire and motivate others for years to come.

Short Success Story 2: Nelson

After being diagnosed with type 2 diabetes, Nelson made a commitment to take control of his health. He worked closely with his healthcare team to develop a plan that included dietary changes, regular exercise, and medication management.

Nelson made a conscious effort to avoid sugary foods and instead focused on eating a nutrient-rich diet with plenty of fruits, vegetables, and lean proteins. He also incorporated regular exercise into his routine, such as walking or biking for 30 minutes a day.

Over time, Nelson's blood sugar levels improved, and he began to see the benefits of his efforts. His energy levels increased, and he felt more in control of his health. Additionally, his healthcare team was able to slowly reduce his medication dosages as his blood sugar levels became more stable.

By making positive lifestyle changes and working closely with his healthcare team, Nelson was able to successfully manage his diabetes and improve his overall health.

Nelson's success in managing his diabetes motivated him to continue making healthy choices. He began to regularly check his blood sugar levels, take his medication on time, and attend regular follow-up appointments with his healthcare team.

He also found support from a local diabetes support group, where he was able to connect with other people who were also managing the condition. This helped him feel less isolated and gave him a sense of community.

As a result of his hard work and dedication, Nelson was able to maintain healthy blood sugar levels and avoid complications from diabetes. He even lost some weight and had more energy to enjoy his favorite activities, such as hiking and playing with his grandchildren.

Nelson's success story is a testament to the power of making positive changes and seeking support in managing chronic conditions. By staying committed to his health and working collaboratively with his healthcare team, he was able to live a full and healthy life despite having diabetes.

Moreover, Nelson's commitment to his health and success in managing his diabetes also inspired others in his support group. He became a mentor and a source of encouragement to those who were struggling with the condition.

Nelson even started volunteering his time to speak at local events to raise awareness about diabetes and inspire others to take control of their health. He became a true advocate for diabetes management and an inspiration to many.

Nelson realized that managing diabetes was not just about taking medication and maintaining healthy habits. It was also about building a community of support and inspiring others to take control of their health. Through his journey, Nelson learned that anyone could thrive with diabetes with the right mindset, support, and commitment.

In the end, Nelson's success in managing his diabetes not only improved his own life but also had a positive impact on his community.

It served as a reminder that chronic conditions like diabetes can be managed effectively with the right approach and support. Nelson's story uplifted the spirits of those who may have considered their condition as a source of shame, guilt, or frustration, empowering them to take control of their lives and health.

Nelson's success story is a beacon of hope for anyone who is struggling with diabetes or any chronic illness. It serves as a testament to the power of positive thinking, the importance of a supportive community, and the role of personal responsibility in managing one's health.

Nelson's journey is proof that with the proper education, resources, and mindset, anyone can live a happy, healthy, and fulfilling life, even with a chronic condition like diabetes.

Furthermore, Nelson's story highlights the importance of seeking out support groups and communities. Having a support system can make all the difference in managing a chronic illness. It can provide emotional support, practical advice, and motivation to stay committed to one's health.

Nelson's commitment to helping others and raising awareness about diabetes also highlights the importance of advocacy. By sharing his story and speaking out about diabetes, Nelson not only helped individuals with the condition but also raised awareness and educated others about the realities of diabetes.

In conclusion, Nelson's journey is a testament to the power of resilience, determination, and community support for managing chronic illness. His story provides hope and inspiration to anyone struggling with health challenges, reminding us that with the right approach, mindset, and support, anything is possible.

It is important to remember that managing a chronic illness like diabetes is not a solo journey. Seeking out resources and support, such as from a healthcare provider or a support group, can have a significant impact on a person's ability to manage their condition and achieve their health goals.

Nelson also exemplifies the importance of self-care. He took responsibility for his own health by making lifestyle changes and staying committed to his treatment plan. By prioritizing self-care, individuals with chronic illness can improve their quality of life and reduce the risk of complications.

Overall, Nelson's story serves as an inspiration to many and highlights the importance of advocacy, community support, and self-care in managing chronic illness. It is a reminder that with determination, education, and support, individuals can overcome challenges and thrive, regardless of their health conditions.

We can reiterate the importance of seeking support and resources for managing chronic illness. It is essential to have regular check-ups with healthcare providers and follow their recommended treatment plans. It is also important to engage in self-care practices, such as healthy eating, regular exercise, stress management, and good sleep habits, to manage the symptoms of chronic illness and improve overall health.

In addition, one may seek out communities and support groups dedicated to individuals with similar health conditions. These groups can offer emotional support, practical advice, and opportunities to learn from others' experiences. By creating a network of support and resources, anyone struggling with a chronic illness can feel less alone, more empowered, and better equipped to manage their condition.

Nelson's story highlights the importance of advocacy and raising awareness about chronic illness. By sharing his story, he motivated others to take control of their health and educated others about the realities of living with diabetes. By becoming advocates, individuals can help raise awareness, break down stigma, and promote better education and resources for managing chronic illness.

In conclusion, managing a chronic illness like diabetes requires a comprehensive approach that includes medical care, self-care, community support, and advocacy. With the right mindset and access to resources, anyone can overcome the challenges of living with a chronic illness and lead a fulfilling life.

Short Success Story 3: Avery

One success story about diabetes is that of a woman named Avery. Avery was diagnosed with type 2 diabetes several years ago and struggled to maintain good blood sugar control, despite following her doctor's recommendations.

Feeling frustrated and discouraged, Avery decided to take matters into her own hands. She began researching diabetes management strategies and implementing lifestyle changes on her own. She started exercising regularly, following a consistent meal plan, and tracking her blood sugar levels closely.

Over time, Avery's dedication and hard work paid off. Her blood sugar levels started to stabilize, and she was able to reduce her reliance on medication. She also started feeling more energetic and confident about her ability to manage her diabetes.

Today, Avery is in better health than ever before. She continues to prioritize her health, living an active lifestyle, and eating a nutritious diet. She also gives back to her community by volunteering with diabetes support groups and spreading awareness about the condition.

Avery's success story is a reminder that with the right mindset, education, and support, it is possible to overcome the challenges of living with diabetes and lead a fulfilling life.

Avery's success story is a true testament to the power of self-care and determination. She not only made significant lifestyle changes to improve her health, but she also became an advocate for diabetes awareness and management.

Through her work with diabetes support groups and awareness campaigns, Avery has inspired countless others to take control of their health and manage their diabetes with confidence. She has even developed a website and blog to share her knowledge and experience with others who are struggling with the condition.

In addition to her community work, Avery also continues to prioritize her own health. She regularly sees her doctor, checks her blood sugar levels, and adjusts her diet and exercise routine as needed. She has also surrounded herself with a supportive network of friends and family members who encourage and uplift her on her journey.

Avery's success story reminds us that a diabetes diagnosis doesn't have to be a life sentence. By taking a proactive approach to self-care and seeking out the best possible resources and support, anyone can overcome the challenges of living with this condition and lead a happy, healthy, and fulfilling life.

Avery's success story is one of resilience, hard work, and determination. When she was diagnosed with diabetes, she knew that she had to take action to manage her health effectively. She made significant changes to her diet and exercise routine, and she worked with her doctor to develop a comprehensive treatment plan that worked for her.

Despite some setbacks and challenges along the way, Avery never let her diagnosis defeat her. She remained focused on her goals and continued to make progress towards better health each day. Over time, her efforts paid off, and she was able to maintain stable blood sugar levels and avoid the complications often associated with diabetes.

But Avery didn't stop there. She channeled her experiences and newfound knowledge into advocating for diabetes awareness and education. She joined a support group and began speaking publicly about her journey, sharing tips and insights with others who were struggling with the condition.

As her message spread, Avery became an inspiration to many. She showed the world that living with diabetes doesn't have to be a burden, and that it's possible to lead a happy and fulfilling life with this condition. Her story inspired others to take control of their health and seek out the resources and support they need to succeed.

Today, Avery continues to be an active advocate for diabetes education and awareness. She has built a strong community of supporters around her, and she takes pride in helping others live healthier, happier lives. Her legacy serves as a reminder that with hard work, dedication, and a positive attitude, anything is possible.

Short Success Story 4: Cruz

Cruz, a 55-year-old man, was diagnosed with type 2 diabetes six years ago. At the time of diagnosis, Cruz's blood sugar level was quite high, and he was overweight, with a BMI of 32. Cruz's doctor advised him to make lifestyle changes, including changes to his diet and exercise habits. Cruz was reluctant to change his habits, but after some encouragement from his family, he finally decided to take action.

Cruz started by monitoring his blood sugar levels regularly, as directed by his doctor. He also made changes to his diet, cutting out processed foods and sugars and eating more fruits and vegetables. Cruz started cooking his meals at home and taking his lunch to work instead of eating fast food. He also started exercising regularly by walking for 30 minutes every day.

After a few weeks of following this new routine, Cruz was surprised to see his blood sugar levels starting to come down. He was feeling more energetic and less lethargic throughout the day. He continued this regimen for the next few months, and his doctor noticed that his blood sugar levels were consistently within the normal range.

Encouraged by his progress, Cruz continued to make lifestyle changes, including joining a support group for people with diabetes. He never missed his regular doctor's appointments and took his medication as prescribed. After a year, Cruz's BMI had dropped to 25, and he had lost 50 pounds. He was no longer on medication and had successfully managed his diabetes through lifestyle changes.

Today, six years after his diagnosis, Cruz is still managing his diabetes successfully. He has maintained a healthy weight, exercises regularly, and eats a balanced diet. Cruz's success story is an inspiration to others who are dealing with diabetes and shows that with the right attitude and lifestyle changes, diabetes can be managed successfully.

Short Success Story 5: Baker

Baker, a 38-year-old mother of two, was diagnosed with type 2 diabetes three years ago. She was shocked when her doctor told her, as she had always considered herself a healthy and active person. However, her diet consisted mostly of processed food and sugary drinks, and her busy schedule left little time for exercise.

After her diagnosis, Baker knew she needed to make significant changes to her lifestyle. She started by consulting a dietitian, who helped her create a healthy meal plan based on whole, unprocessed foods and lean protein sources. Baker also stopped drinking sugary beverages and switched to water and herbal tea.

To increase her physical activity, Baker started walking for 30 minutes every day, gradually increasing the duration and intensity of her workouts. She also started lifting weights to build muscle and boost her metabolism.

With time and dedication, Baker's efforts paid off. Her blood sugar levels began to normalize, and her doctor started lowering her medication dosage. She also noticed that she had more energy and felt better overall.

Encouraged by her progress, Baker continued to implement healthy habits into her daily routine. She joined a support group for people with diabetes, which provided her with emotional support and helped her stay motivated.

Today, three years later, Baker's diabetes is under control, and she no longer requires medication. She has lost weight, improved her fitness level, and feels better than she ever has. Baker's success story is a testament to the power of lifestyle changes in managing diabetes and achieving better health.

Short Success Story 6: Simon

Simon, a 55-year-old man, was diagnosed with type 2 diabetes 15 years ago. He struggled to manage his blood sugar levels for years, relying heavily on medication and insulin injections.

However, after a health scare that left him hospitalized, Simon knew he needed to make a drastic change. He reached out to a diabetes educator who helped him create a personalized plan to manage his diabetes.

Simon started by overhauling his diet, cutting out processed foods, sugary drinks, and refined carbohydrates. He began eating whole, nutrient-dense foods, including lean proteins, vegetables, and complex carbohydrates. He also started tracking his meals to ensure he was getting the right balance of macronutrients.

In addition to improving his diet, Simon started incorporating exercise into his daily routine. He began with short walks and gradually increased the duration and intensity of his workouts. He also started doing resistance training to build muscle mass and boost his metabolism.

With time and consistency, Simon's blood sugar levels began to stabilize. His doctor gradually reduced his medication dosage until he no longer needed insulin injections. Simon also started to notice other health benefits, such as improved energy levels, better sleep, and a stronger immune system.

Today, Simon continues to manage his diabetes through a healthy diet and regular exercise. He has maintained a healthy weight, and his blood sugar levels have remained stable for several years. Simon's success story shows that with dedication and hard work, it is possible to manage diabetes and achieve better overall health.

Short Success Story 7: Maria

Maria, a 42-year-old woman, was diagnosed with type 2 diabetes five years ago. She was initially in denial and struggled to come to terms with her diagnosis. However, after experiencing several health complications related to diabetes, Maria knew she needed to take control of her health.

She started by consulting a dietitian who helped her create a healthy meal plan based on whole, unprocessed foods. Maria also started tracking her food intake and blood sugar levels, which helped her identify patterns and make adjustments to her diet.

Maria also began a regular exercise routine, which included a combination of cardio and strength training. She started slowly with low-impact exercises like walking and yoga and gradually built up to more intense workouts.

Over time, Maria's hard work paid off. Her blood sugar levels stabilized, and she was able to reduce her medication dosage. She also noticed other health benefits, such as improved energy levels and better sleep.

Encouraged by her progress, Maria started advocating for diabetes awareness and education in her community. She shared her story and encouraged others to make healthy lifestyle changes manage their diabetes.

Today, Maria is still managing her diabetes through a healthy diet and regular exercise. She has also joined a support group for people with diabetes, where she can connect with others and share her experiences. Maria's success story shows that with dedication and commitment, it is possible to manage diabetes and improve overall health.

Short Success Story 8: Liam

Liam, a 37-year-old man, was diagnosed with type 2 diabetes eight years ago. He struggled to manage his condition, relying heavily on medication and feeling disheartened by the constant blood sugar fluctuations.

One day, a friend introduced Liam to the concept of a low-carbohydrate diet. Liam was skeptical at first, but after doing some research and talking to his doctor, he decided to give it a try.

Liam overhauled his diet, eliminating processed and high-carbohydrate foods and replacing them with healthy fats, proteins, and non-starchy vegetables. He also started tracking his food intake and blood sugar levels to monitor his progress.

At first, it was difficult for Liam to adjust to his new diet. But over time, he started to notice significant improvements in his blood sugar levels. His medication dosage was gradually reduced, and soon he was able to stop taking medication altogether.

Emboldened by his success, Liam started to incorporate more exercise into his routine, focusing on strength training and high-intensity interval training (HIIT). He found that regular exercise helped to further stabilize his blood sugar levels and improve his overall health.

Today, Liam has maintained his low-carbohydrate diet and regular exercise routine for several years with great success. His blood sugar levels remain stable, and he no longer needs medication to manage his diabetes. Liam's success story shows that with determination and a willingness to try new things, it is possible to overcome diabetes and reclaim one's health.

Short Success Story 9: Anita

Anita, a 52-year-old woman, was diagnosed with type 2 diabetes 12 years ago. For years, she struggled to manage her condition, relying heavily on medication and feeling hopeless about her health.

One day, Anita's daughter encouraged her to try a plant-based diet. Anita was skeptical at first, as she was used to eating meat and dairy regularly. However, she decided to give it a try.

Anita transitioned to a plant-based diet gradually, starting by incorporating more fruits, vegetables, and whole grains into her meals. She also started tracking her food intake and blood sugar levels, which helped her understand how different foods affected her health.

Over time, Anita noticed significant improvements in her blood sugar levels. She was able to reduce her medication dosage and eventually, stop taking medication altogether. She also experienced other health benefits, such as improved digestion and more energy.

Buoyed by her success, Anita started to incorporate more physical activity into her routine. She started by going for daily walks and gradually built up to more intense workouts, such as yoga and Pilates.

Today, Anita is still managing her diabetes through a plant-based diet and regular exercise. She has also become an advocate for plant-based eating and diabetes management in her community. Anita's success story shows that making small changes to one's lifestyle can have a big impact on health and well-being.

Short Success Story 10: Roberto

Roberto, a 45-year-old man, was diagnosed with type 2 diabetes six years ago. Despite taking medication and following his doctor's instructions, he found it difficult to manage his blood sugar levels.

Determined to take control of his health, Roberto started researching alternative ways of managing his diabetes. He stumbled upon a program promoting a high-fat, low-carbohydrate diet, and decided to give it a try.

Roberto eliminated processed and high-carbohydrate foods from his diet, which he found challenging at first. But as he began to incorporate healthy fats such as avocado, nuts and olive oil, he noticed a significant improvement in his blood sugar levels.

Roberto also started weightlifting and doing regular cardiovascular exercise, which further stabilized his blood sugar levels and improved his overall health.

Over time, Roberto was able to reduce his medication dosage and eventually, stop taking medication altogether. Today, he maintains a high-fat, low-carbohydrate diet and an active lifestyle, and manages his diabetes successfully without medication.

Roberto's success story demonstrates that by being proactive, open-minded and making positive lifestyle changes, it is possible to overcome type 2 diabetes and achieve a healthier, more fulfilling life.

Short Success Story 11: Baily

When Bailey was diagnosed with type 2 diabetes at age 47, she was shocked. She had always been conscious of her weight and had eaten a healthy diet, or so she thought.

But after learning more about the disease, Bailey realized that her diet had a lot of hidden sugars, and she also wasn't as active as she thought she was. She decided to make some changes.

Bailey started by tracking her blood sugar levels and keeping a food diary, which helped her identify problem areas in her diet. She then worked with a nutritionist to develop a meal plan that focused on lean protein, whole grains, fruits, and vegetables.

In addition to changing her diet, Bailey started taking daily walks and gradually built up to more intense workouts, like strength training and yoga. With the help of regular exercise and a healthy diet, Bailey was able to lose weight and stabilize her blood sugar levels.

Over time, Bailey's dedication to her health paid off. She was able to stop taking medication and her doctor gave her the green light to only come in for check ups every three months instead of every month like before.

Today, Bailey has maintained her healthy lifestyle and remains symptom-free. Despite the challenges of having type 2 diabetes, Bailey knows that with discipline and perseverance, it's possible to control the disease and live a full, happy life.

Short Success Story 12: Cohen

Cohen was diagnosed with type 2 diabetes at age 58. He had always been a bit overweight and enjoyed eating sugary snacks and drinking soda, but he never realized the impact it was having on his health.

After his diagnosis, Cohen was determined to take control of his health and reverse his diabetes. He started by cutting out all sugary treats and replacing them with healthier options like fruit and nuts.

Cohen also started going for daily walks and eventually joined a gym to do strength training and cardio workouts. As his fitness level improved, he started running and participating in charity races, which helped him stay motivated.

In addition to changing his diet and exercise habits, Cohen started taking supplements and herbs that are known to lower blood sugar levels, like cinnamon and chromium.

Over time, Cohen's commitment to his health paid off. His blood sugar levels became normal and his doctor was amazed at how much his health had improved. Cohen no longer needed medication and was able to maintain his health through diet and exercise alone.

Today, Cohen remains diabetes-free and continues to prioritize his health and fitness. He is grateful for the second chance at life he was given and encourages others with diabetes to take control of their health and never give up hope.

Short Success Story 13: Tony

Tony struggled with weight and blood sugar control for many years before being diagnosed with type 2 diabetes at age 40. She knew she needed to make changes to improve her health, but wasn't sure where to start.

Tony began by educating herself about diabetes and the role that diet and exercise play in managing the disease. She then worked with a nutritionist to develop a meal plan that focused on whole, unprocessed foods and limited added sugars.

In addition to changing her diet, Tony started exercising regularly. She began by going for daily walks and gradually increased the intensity and duration of her workouts over time. She also started practicing stress management techniques like meditation and yoga, which helped her manage her blood sugar levels.

With the support of her family and healthcare team, Tony was able to lose a significant amount of weight and improve her blood sugar control. Her doctor was amazed at her progress and eventually gave her the go-ahead to stop taking her diabetes medication.

Now, Tony continues to prioritize her health by eating a balanced diet, exercising regularly, and practicing stress management techniques. She also works as a diabetes educator, sharing her story and helping others who are struggling with the disease.

Short Success Story 14: David

David was diagnosed with type 2 diabetes when he was in his late 50s. He had a family history of the disease, but he never paid much attention to his diet or exercise habits until he received the diagnosis.

David began by tracking his blood sugar levels and working with a nutritionist to create a meal plan that would help him manage his diabetes. He focused on eating more whole grains, fruits, and vegetables, and started cooking at home more often.

In addition to changing his diet, David started going for daily walks and eventually joined a gym. He worked with a personal trainer to develop strength training and cardio routine that was tailored to his needs.

David also started practicing stress management techniques like deep breathing and mindfulness meditation, which helped him manage his blood sugar levels and improve his overall well-being.

With time and dedication, David was able to successfully manage his diabetes. His blood sugar levels became normal, and he was able to reduce his medication dosage under his doctor's guidance.

Today, David continues to prioritize his health and wellness by following a healthy diet, staying active, and practicing stress management techniques. He is grateful for the support of his family and healthcare team, and encourage others with diabetes to never give up on their health goals.

Short Success Story 15: Ashley

Ashley was diagnosed with type 2 diabetes when she was in her mid-30s. She had always struggled with her weight and had a family history of diabetes, so the diagnosis didn't come as a surprise.

Ashley knew that she needed to make big changes in order to improve her health and manage her diabetes. She began by working with a nutritionist to develop a personalized meal plan that focused on whole, unprocessed foods and limited added sugars.

In addition to changing her diet, Ashley started going for daily walks and eventually joined a fitness class that she enjoyed. She also began incorporating yoga and meditation into her routine to help manage her stress levels.

With time, Ashley was able to lose a significant amount of weight and manage her diabetes with diet and exercise alone. She no longer needed to rely on medication or insulin injections.

Ashley continues to prioritize her health by eating a balanced diet, staying active, and practicing stress management techniques. She has also become an advocate for diabetes awareness and prevention, sharing her story and encouraging others to take control of their health.

Short Success Story 16: Jacob

Jacob was diagnosed with type 2 diabetes when he was in his early 40s. He had a sedentary lifestyle and a diet full of processed and sugary foods, which contributed to his disease.

Jacob knew he needed to make some major changes to his lifestyle in order to manage his diabetes. He began by consulting with a nutritionist to develop a healthy meal plan that focused on fiber-rich foods and lean proteins. He also began cooking more often at home and reduced his intake of processed foods and sugars.

Jacob also started exercising regularly by joining a gym and working with a personal trainer. He began with light cardio and strength training and gradually increased the intensity and duration of his workouts.

As Jacob continued with his healthy diet and exercise routine, he noticed significant improvements in his diabetes management. His blood sugar levels started to stabilize, and he was able to reduce his medication dosage and eventually eliminate it completely under his doctor's guidance.

Today, Jacob continues to maintain his healthy lifestyle by eating a balanced diet, exercising regularly, and monitoring his blood sugar levels. He is grateful for the positive changes he made in his life and encourages others with diabetes to take charge of their health by making similar changes.

Short Success Story 17: Cooper

Cooper was diagnosed with prediabetes in her early 20s. She was initially reluctant to make changes to her lifestyle. However, as she learned more about the serious complications that can arise from mismanaged diabetes, she made a commitment to change her habits.

Cooper began by cutting back on junk food and sugary drinks and instead, focused on eating more fruits, vegetables, and lean proteins. She also started taking regular walks and even signed up for a fun dance fitness class.

With time, Cooper was able to lose weight, reduce her blood sugar levels, and return to a healthy glucose range. Despite facing some setbacks along the way, she remained dedicated to her health and is now able to manage her diabetes with just a few lifestyle changes.

Cooper's experience taught her the importance of staying proactive when it comes to health, and now she encourages others to take the necessary steps toward better diabetes management.

As a result of Cooper's commitment to her health, she not only managed to avoid the most serious complications of diabetes, but also regained her confidence and energy levels. She was able to pursue her career with renewed focus and enthusiasm, and even found time to volunteer for local diabetes advocacy groups. The changes she made to her lifestyle not only allowed her to thrive with diabetes, but also improved her overall quality of life. Cooper's success story serves as an inspiration to others facing similar health challenges, and reminds us of the power of diet, exercise, and positive habits on our well-being.

Furthermore, Cooper's dedication to her health did not just benefit herself, but also those around her. Her family and friends were amazed by her transformation and were inspired by her perseverance. She started to share her journey with others, offering support and encouragement to those who were struggling with similar health challenges. Cooper's positive attitude and resilience became contagious, creating a ripple effect of healthy habits and positive lifestyle changes in her community.

Cooper's story is a testament to the fact that managing diabetes is not just about taking medications, but also about making lifestyle changes to promote long-term health. With the right diet, exercise, and mindset, it is possible to not only manage diabetes, but also improve overall health and well-being. Cooper's journey shows that with commitment and determination, anything is possible, and that a diagnosis of diabetes does not have to define one's life.

Moreover, Cooper's involvement in diabetes advocacy groups allowed her to make a difference in the lives of others affected by the condition. Through her volunteer work, she was able to raise awareness about diabetes and promote education in healthy lifestyle changes. She became a role model for those who were struggling to manage their diabetes, showing them that it was possible to live a fulfilling life with the condition.

Cooper's story also highlights the importance of early diagnosis and proactive management of diabetes. By taking an active role in managing her health, Cooper was able to prevent serious complications and maintain a high quality of life. Her story serves as a reminder that taking small, consistent steps towards better health can have a significant impact on our overall well-being.

In conclusion, Cooper's success story is a testament to the power of determination and positive lifestyle changes in managing diabetes. Her journey should serve as an inspiration to anyone facing similar health challenges, and a reminder that with the right mindset and support, it is possible to live a healthy and fulfilling life, even with a chronic condition.

We can recognize the significance of her journey in raising awareness about diabetes and promoting healthy living. Cooper's story shows that through dedication, perseverance, and a positive attitude, individuals can take control of their diabetes and improve their overall health and well-being. Her involvement in diabetes advocacy groups is a remarkable example of how individuals can work together to create positive change and make a difference in the lives of others.

Additionally, Cooper's story highlights the importance of taking proactive measures when managing chronic conditions like diabetes. By keeping a healthy diet, exercising regularly, and monitoring her blood sugar levels, Cooper was able to prevent the development of serious health complications and maintain a good quality of life. Her journey serves as an inspiration to others to take control of their health and make positive lifestyle changes manage their conditions.

Finally, Cooper's involvement in advocacy groups shows how important it is to raise awareness about diabetes and other chronic conditions. Her efforts in promoting education on healthy lifestyle changes and raising awareness about diabetes have helped to reduce the stigma associated with the condition. Her story serves as a reminder that with the right mindset and support, individuals with chronic conditions can lead fulfilling and successful lives.

However, I recognize the significance of Cooper's story in promoting the importance of healthy lifestyle choices and self-care for individuals with chronic conditions like diabetes. Her journey serves as an inspiration for those who may be struggling with their own health, showing that with dedication and positivity, it is possible to lead a fulfilling life and make a positive impact on the world.

Cooper's story not only shows the importance of managing chronic conditions through healthy lifestyle habits, but also highlights the impact that advocacy and raising awareness can have in improving the lives of those with similar conditions. Her journey serves as a motivation for individuals to take proactive measures to manage their health and to become advocates for their own conditions, and to inspire others to make positive changes for themselves as well.

Yes, absolutely. It's essential to take control of our own health and to be proactive in managing any chronic conditions we may have. By following healthy lifestyle habits such as eating a balanced diet, getting regular exercise, and practicing self-care, we can make a significant impact on our physical and mental well-being. And as you said, by sharing our stories and advocating for our own conditions, we can raise awareness and help others who may be going through similar struggles. Cooper's journey is a perfect example of this, and her success should encourage us to take a similar proactive approach to promote our own health and advocating for important causes.

Short Success Story 18: Gary

One inspiring success story about managing diabetes is that of Gary Hall Jr. He was diagnosed with type 1 diabetes at the age of 25, which could have ended his career as an Olympic swimmer. However, he refused to let diabetes be a barrier to his athletic dreams and became an advocate for diabetes management.

Gary worked with a team of doctors to develop a strict health management plan, which included a healthy diet, regular exercise, and constant monitoring of his blood sugar levels. He went on to win 10 Olympic medals and continued to inspire others with diabetes to pursue their dreams and lead healthy lifestyles.

Today, Gary is still an active advocate for diabetes management and has co-founded the organization, Insulindependence, which promotes active lifestyles and community support for those living with diabetes. His story serves as a powerful reminder that with dedication, discipline, and proper management, diabetes can be managed, and dreams can still be achieved.

Gary's dedication to diabetes management and advocacy did not end with his Olympic career. He continued to use his platform and voice to raise awareness and support for those living with diabetes. In 2012, he joined forces with the Diabetes Research Institute Foundation to launch the "Athletes for a Cure" campaign, which aimed to raise funds for diabetes research and to inspire those living with diabetes to lead active and healthy lifestyles.

Gary's success story highlights the importance of proper diabetes management, which can not only improve the quality of life for those living with diabetes but also help them achieve their dreams. Through his advocacy and example, Gary has shown that diabetes does not have to be a limitation, and with the right support, anyone can live a fulfilling and active life.

Gary's passion for the cause was driven by his own experiences of living with diabetes. He knew firsthand the challenges and struggles that come with managing the condition, from constantly monitoring blood sugar levels to carefully planning meals and exercise routines. Yet, he refused to let diabetes hold him back.

Gary believed that education and awareness were key to overcoming the stigma and misconceptions surrounding diabetes. He spoke openly about his own experiences, sharing tips and advice on managing diabetes while pursuing an athletic career. He also used his platform to raise awareness and funds for diabetes research, hoping to someday find a cure for this chronic condition.

Today, Gary's legacy lives on through the many lives he touched and inspired. His dedication to diabetes management and advocacy has made a significant impact in the diabetes community, and his story continues to inspire others to never give up on their dreams, no matter what challenges they may face.

Gary's story reminds us that living with diabetes does not have to limit our lives. With proper management, support, and advocacy, we can overcome the challenges of this condition and achieve our goals. His dedication and advocacy have helped to break down the stigma associated with diabetes and inspire others to take control of their health. He has left a lasting impact on the diabetes community, and his legacy will continue to inspire future generations.

Gary's journey with diabetes began when he was just a child. At the age of 10, he was diagnosed with type 1 diabetes, a chronic condition that requires constant monitoring and management. Growing up, he faced many challenges, including the stigma associated with diabetes and the social isolation that often comes with the condition.

Despite the challenges, Gary was determined not to let diabetes limit his life. He embraced a healthy lifestyle, including regular exercise and a balanced diet. He also became an advocate for diabetes awareness and education, working with organizations like the American Diabetes Association and JDRF to raise awareness about the condition and support research for a cure.

In his adult years, Gary's advocacy efforts became even more prominent. He began speaking out publicly about his experience with diabetes, sharing his story with others and encouraging them to take control of their health. He also worked to break down the myths and misconceptions surrounding diabetes, helping others understand that it is a manageable condition that doesn't have to limit their lives.

Through it all, Gary served as an inspiration to countless people living with diabetes. His dedication and advocacy efforts helped to improve the quality of life for those with the condition, and his legacy continues to inspire people today. Although Gary is no longer with us, his impact on the diabetes community will be felt for years to come.

Short Success Story 19: Lisa

Lisa was diagnosed with Type 2 Diabetes when she was only 30 years old. She was devastated and struggled to cope with the diagnosis as she felt like her life was over.

Lisa decided to take the bull by the horns and make the best of her situation. She met with a certified diabetes educator who taught her about the disease, how to manage it with diet and exercise, and how to test her blood sugar.

Lisa made a plan for herself that included regular exercise, a healthy and balanced diet, and monitoring her blood sugar levels. Within just a few months, she started to see results. Her blood sugar levels were lower, she had lost weight, and her energy levels had increased.

Through hard work and discipline, Lisa was able to completely reverse her diabetes. She went from being dependent on insulin to being medication-free in just six months.

Lisa became an advocate for diabetes prevention and management, sharing her experience with others who were struggling with the disease. She encouraged others to take their diabetes seriously, make lifestyle changes, and control their diabetes.

Today, Lisa is living a happy and healthy life, free from the burdens of diabetes. She feels fortunate to have experienced this journey of self-discovery, and is grateful for the support of family, friends and medical professionals who helped her along the way.

Lisa's success story spread quickly, and many people started reaching out to her for advice and guidance on managing their diabetes. She started organizing workshops and seminars in her community to raise awareness and educate people about the disease.

Lisa's efforts paid off, and many individuals were able to successfully manage their diabetes. She even received an award from a local organization for her achievements in diabetes advocacy.

But Lisa didn't stop there. She realized that there were many people who couldn't afford diabetes medication or didn't have access to proper healthcare. She started a non-profit organization to help such individuals, providing them with free diabetes education, medication, and support.

Her organization's efforts have helped thousands of people, and Lisa's story continues to inspire many across the world. The impact she has made on the lives of people affected by diabetes is immeasurable, and her dedication to helping others is an inspiration to all.

Short Success Story 20: Kennedy

After being diagnosed with diabetes, Kennedy made a commitment to take control of his health. He began monitoring his blood sugar levels regularly, eating a balanced diet and exercising regularly. It was challenging, but he refused to let his diagnosis define him.

Over time, Kennedy's dedication paid off. His blood sugar levels stabilized, his energy levels increased, and he lost weight. His doctor was so impressed that he was able to reduce Kennedy's medication dosage.

Encouraged by his progress, Kennedy started sharing his journey with others. He joined a local support group and began volunteering at diabetes awareness events. He also started a blog to document his experiences and give advice to others living with diabetes.

As Kennedy's knowledge and experience grew, so did his impact. He became a trusted advocate for diabetes awareness and management in his community, and his blog gained a large following.

Even though diabetes will always be a part of Kennedy's life, he refuses to be defined by it. Through his hard work and perseverance, he has become a successful voice for diabetes awareness and a source of hope for others facing a similar journey.

However, I've learned that maintaining a healthy lifestyle can control blood sugar levels effectively. People with diabetes can lead a fulfilling life by following their doctor's advice and making lifestyle changes. Like Kennedy, they can be a valuable part of their community by sharing their experiences and inspiring others to take control of their health.

One day, Kennedy encountered a young boy who had just been diagnosed with type 1 diabetes. The boy was scared and did not understand what was happening to him. Kennedy stopped and talked to the boy and his parents, explaining that he also had diabetes and that it was possible to live a healthy life with the condition.

Kennedy showed the boy how to check his blood sugar levels and how to properly administer insulin. He also shared with the family resources and information on diabetes education and support groups. The boy and his parents left feeling more informed and less anxious about their new reality.

Kennedy felt happy knowing that he was able to help someone else going through what he had experienced. He continued to be an advocate for diabetes awareness and education, always willing to share his story and knowledge with others who needed it.

Years later, Kennedy was honored by the American Diabetes Association for his work as an advocate for diabetes awareness and education. He continued his work, knowing that there were still many people who needed support and information to manage their diabetes effectively. Kennedy's dedication and commitment to others with diabetes had made a positive impact on their lives and had also enriched his own journey with the condition.

As Kennedy got older, he faced new challenges with diabetes. He struggled with neuropathy, a nerve condition that caused numbness and tingling in his feet. He also had to manage his blood pressure and cholesterol levels to lower his risk of heart disease, a common complication of diabetes.

Despite these challenges, Kennedy remained determined to live the best life he could with diabetes. He adapted his exercise routine to include low-impact activities, such as swimming and yoga. He also made healthy diet choices and took his medication as prescribed.

Kennedy continued to inspire others with diabetes by sharing his own struggles and strategies for managing the condition. He spoke at conferences and wrote articles for diabetes publications. He also volunteered with diabetes advocacy groups and served as a mentor to newly diagnosed individuals.

In his later years, Kennedy faced additional health challenges and eventually passed away at the age of 80. However, his legacy as a diabetes advocate and voice of encouragement lived on. He had touched countless lives with his kindness, generosity, and passion for helping others live well with diabetes.

In honor of Kennedy's dedication to helping others with diabetes, his family established a foundation in his name to support diabetes research and education. The foundation raised funds to support local diabetes clinics, provide scholarships for diabetes education programs, and sponsor community awareness events.

Kennedy's impact on the diabetes community continued to grow even after his passing. His story was shared in diabetes publications and online forums, inspiring others with the condition to live their best lives and advocate for their health.

Thanks to Kennedy's advocacy and the work of countless others, awareness and understanding of diabetes continued to improve over the years. New treatment options, technologies, and lifestyle management strategies were developed to help people with diabetes live healthy and fulfilling lives.

Kennedy's legacy as a diabetes advocate and champion will always be remembered and honored by the many lives he touched during his lifetime.

The Kennedy Diabetes Foundation became a pillar of the diabetes community, providing resources and support for those affected by the condition. Its impact extended far beyond its local community, reaching people around the world through its online resources and partnerships with international diabetes organizations.

Through the foundation, Kennedy's family continued his legacy of advocacy, dedicating themselves to raising awareness about diabetes and working to improve the lives of those affected by the condition.

As the years went by, the foundation continued to grow and evolve, always staying true to Kennedy's vision of empowering people with diabetes to live their best lives. It provided grants for diabetes research, supported the development of new technologies and treatments, and advocated for improved access to diabetes care for all.

Through it all, Kennedy's unwavering spirit and passion for helping others with diabetes remained a driving force for the foundation, inspiring everyone involved working harder and dream bigger.

Thanks to Kennedy's legacy and the tireless efforts of the Kennedy Diabetes Foundation, diabetes was no longer seen as a barrier to living a full and rewarding life. It was simply a challenge to be faced head-on, with strength, determination, and the support of a caring community.

The foundation's impact was felt in countless ways, from the families who received support and education through its programs to the researchers who received funding for groundbreaking studies that helped unlock new treatments and therapies for diabetes.

Kennedy's family worked tirelessly to ensure that his legacy would continue to be felt for generations to come. They continued to raise funds and awareness for the foundation, inspiring others to join the fight against diabetes and giving hope to those affected by the condition.

Thanks to their dedication and the countless others who contributed to the foundation's success, Kennedy's dream of a world where diabetes was no longer a barrier to living a full and healthy life became a reality.

And while Kennedy may no longer be with us, his legacy of advocacy, compassion, and tireless dedication to helping others with diabetes will continue to inspire and empower people around the world for years to come.

The Kennedy Diabetes Foundation became a beacon of hope for those affected by diabetes, providing a supportive community and vital resources to help manage the condition and improve quality of life.

The foundation's impact was far-reaching, with its programs and initiatives helping people around the world access the tools and information needed to live well with diabetes. Its partnerships with other organizations and researchers also helped advance the field of diabetes research and treatment, leading to breakthroughs that changed the lives of millions.

Through it all, Kennedy's family remained committed to his vision and worked tirelessly to ensure that the foundation continued to make a difference in the lives of those affected by diabetes. They knew that Kennedy's legacy was too important to let fade away, and so they carried on his mission with the same passion and determination that he had embodied.

Thanks to their efforts and the support of the diabetes community, the Kennedy Diabetes Foundation will continue to be a force for good in the fight against diabetes for years to come. And although Kennedy may no longer be with us, his spirit lives on in the foundation he created and the lives that he touched.

The impact of the Kennedy Diabetes Foundation has been immeasurable, and its contributions to the diabetes community will be felt for generations. The foundation's legacy serves as a testament to the power of advocacy, compassion, and determination in the face of adversity.

Kennedy's vision of a world where diabetes is no longer a barrier to living a full and healthy life has become a reality in many ways, thanks to the work of the foundation and the diabetes community at large. With continued support and collaboration, there is hope that a cure for diabetes may one day be within reach.

For everyone who has been touched by diabetes, the Kennedy Diabetes Foundation will always be a symbol of hope and a source of inspiration. Its mission to improve the lives of those with diabetes, to support research and education, and to advocate for change will continue to shape the world in the years to come.

The foundation's impact has been felt globally, with its programs and initiatives reaching people across continents and cultures. Through its advocacy efforts, the foundation has worked to raise awareness about diabetes and the challenges faced by those living with the condition. By promoting education and providing access to resources, the foundation has helped individuals better manage their diabetes and improve their quality of life.

One of the most significant accomplishments of the Kennedy Diabetes Foundation has been its support for diabetes research. By funding cutting-edge research and partnering with leading experts in the field, the foundation has helped advance our understanding of diabetes and develop new treatments and therapies. This work has led to breakthroughs that have transformed the lives of those living with diabetes, and it holds promise for continued progress in the future.

Despite the foundation's many successes, there is still much work to be done. Diabetes remains a significant health challenge, affecting millions of people around the world. By continuing to support research, education, and advocacy, the Kennedy Diabetes Foundation can help pave the way toward better treatment and ultimately, a cure. And in doing so, it will continue to honor the legacy of Kennedy and his vision for a world free of the barriers imposed by diabetes.

The foundation's impact can also be seen through the support it provides to individuals with diabetes and their families. Through its programs and resources, the foundation has helped individuals better understand and manage their condition, while also offering emotional and practical support. This support has been invaluable in helping individuals with diabetes lead full and fulfilling lives, despite the challenges of the condition.

In addition, the foundation's focus on advocacy has helped bring attention to the social and economic factors that contribute to diabetes prevalence and hinder access to care. By advocating for policy changes and increased resources for diabetes prevention and treatment, the foundation has helped address key barriers to care and improve health outcomes for those with diabetes.

Overall, the Kennedy Diabetes Foundation has had a profound impact on the diabetes community and beyond.

Through its unwavering commitment to improving the lives of those with diabetes, advancing scientific knowledge, and advocating for change, the foundation has helped shape a brighter future for individuals with diabetes and their families. Its legacy will continue to inspire and guide the diabetes community in their efforts to overcome the challenges of the condition and work towards a cure.

The foundation has also played a significant role in promoting diabetes prevention and early detection. By emphasizing the importance of healthy eating and physical activity, as well as regular screenings and check-ups, the foundation has helped individuals reduce their risk of developing diabetes or catch the condition early when it is most treatable. This approach has a ripple effect, as individuals are able to take control of their health and prevent or minimize the impact of diabetes on their lives.

Another notable achievement of the Kennedy Diabetes Foundation is its efforts to build partnerships and collaborations across fields and sectors. By bringing together experts from different disciplines and organizations, the foundation has been able to leverage diverse perspectives and resources to advance its mission. This approach has been particularly effective in supporting diabetes research, as the foundation has been able to attract top talent and foster innovation through its network of collaborators.

Looking to the future, the Kennedy Diabetes Foundation will undoubtedly continue to make a significant impact in the fight against diabetes. Whether through advocacy, education, research, or support for individuals and families affected by diabetes, the foundation will remain a beacon of hope and progress in the diabetes community and beyond. With its strong leadership, strategic vision, and unwavering commitment to its mission, the foundation is poised to make even greater strides in improving the lives of those with diabetes and ultimately finding a cure for the condition.

The foundation has also been instrumental in raising awareness about the global burden of diabetes. Through its international partnerships and collaborations, the foundation has helped shine a spotlight on the disparities in diabetes prevalence and access to care around the world. The foundation has also supported initiatives to promote diabetes prevention and management in low- and middle-income countries, where the burden of the condition is often greatest.

In addition to its advocacy and support for research, the Kennedy Diabetes Foundation has also invested in technological innovations that hold promise for improving diabetes care. For example, the foundation has supported the development of digital health tools, such as mobile apps and wearable devices that can help individuals with diabetes monitor their blood glucose levels, track their food intake and physical activity, and manage their medications. These tools can help individuals better manage their condition and empower them to take control of their health.

Overall, the Kennedy Diabetes Foundation has made an indelible mark on the diabetes community and the broader public health landscape. By championing research, education, advocacy, support, and innovation, the foundation has helped millions of individuals with diabetes around the world lead healthier and more fulfilling lives. As the foundation continues its work, it will undoubtedly inspire others to join the fight against diabetes and work towards a future where the condition is a thing of the past.

Short Success Story 21: Mary

One success story about diabetes is that of a woman named Mary, who was diagnosed with type 2 diabetes in her early 40s. At the time of her diagnosis, Mary was overweight and her blood sugar levels were consistently high. She was prescribed medication and advised making significant lifestyle changes manage her condition.

Over the next few years, Mary worked with a diabetes educator and a nutritionist to improve her diet and increase her physical activity. She started taking regular walks and began incorporating more fruits, vegetables, and whole grains into her meals. She also learned how to monitor her blood glucose levels at home and made adjustments to her medication as needed.

Through hard work and dedication, Mary was able to achieve significant improvements in her health. She lost over 50 pounds and her blood sugar levels stabilized within a healthy range. She was eventually able to reduce her medication dosage and her doctor indicated that she may be able to stop taking medication altogether in the future.

Today, Mary continues to manage her diabetes through a healthy diet and regular exercise. She has become an advocate for diabetes awareness and speaks to others about the importance of early detection and proactive management. Mary's story is a testament to the fact that with the right support, knowledge, and determination, it is possible to successfully manage diabetes and live a healthy, fulfilling life.

Mary's success story did not end with achieving better health and becoming an advocate for diabetes awareness. After her own experience with diabetes, Mary went back to school to become a certified diabetes educator herself. She wanted to use her own experience and knowledge to help others living with diabetes navigate the challenges of managing their condition.

Now, as a certified diabetes educator, Mary works with individuals and groups to help them develop personalized strategies for managing their diabetes. She emphasizes the importance of building a support system, setting goals, and taking small but consistent steps towards better health. Mary also advocates for greater access to diabetes education and resources for underserved communities.

Mary's tireless work and dedication to diabetes management and advocacy have earned her recognition and awards from various organizations. She has been featured in numerous media outlets, sharing her story and spreading awareness about diabetes.

Mary's journey is a true testament to the power of determination, hard work, and the importance of receiving support and guidance in managing diabetes. Her success story demonstrates that with the right tools and mindset, it is possible to thrive despite a diabetes diagnosis.

In addition to her work as a certified diabetes educator, Mary also became involved in diabetes research. She co-authored several studies on the impact of diabetes on mental health and the benefits of mindfulness-based interventions for individuals with diabetes.

Mary's passion for diabetes management and advocacy continued to grow, and she eventually started her own nonprofit organization focused on diabetes education and support. The organization provides resources and guidance to individuals and families affected by diabetes, as well as organizes community events and outreach programs.

Through her work as a diabetes educator, researcher, and nonprofit founder, Mary has helped countless individuals with diabetes live healthier, happier lives. Her dedication to diabetes management and advocacy has made a significant impact on the diabetes community, and her success story serves as an inspiration to others living with diabetes.

Mary's achievements did not go unnoticed. She was invited to speak at conferences and events, both nationally and internationally, about her work and the importance of diabetes education and advocacy. Her speaking engagements allowed her to reach even more people with her message, and she became a sought-after voice in the diabetes community.

Through all of her accomplishments, Mary never lost sight of her own journey with diabetes. She continues to manage her condition with a positive and proactive mindset, and uses her personal experiences as inspiration for her advocacy and educational work.

Mary's story shows that a diabetes diagnosis does not have to be the end of a fulfilling and happy life. With the right mindset, support, and education, it is possible to not only manage diabetes, but to thrive and make a difference in the world. Mary serves as a shining example of this, and her dedication to improving the lives of those living with diabetes is truly inspiring.

As Mary's nonprofit organization continued to grow, she expanded its reach by launching an online platform that offers resources and support to individuals with diabetes around the world. The platform provides access to educational materials, webinars, and peer support groups, as well as a directory of diabetes care providers and resources.

Through her organization and online platform, Mary has created a community of individuals with diabetes, who support each other in their journey of managing the condition. Mary also advocates for diabetes education and access to care at the policy level, working with lawmakers to ensure that individuals with diabetes have the support and resources they need to live healthy and fulfilling lives.

Mary's contributions to the diabetes community have been recognized with numerous awards and honors, including the American Diabetes Association's Outstanding Educator in Diabetes Award and the Juvenile Diabetes Research Foundation's Humanitarian of the Year Award.

Mary's story is a testament to the power of perseverance and advocacy in overcoming the challenges of living with a chronic condition. She has used her personal experience to help countless others with diabetes, and her legacy will continue to inspire future generations of diabetes educators and advocates.

Mary's tireless efforts and advocacy has truly made a difference in the lives of people with diabetes. Through her educational programs, online platform, and policy work, she has helped individuals gain the knowledge and resources they need to manage their condition and live healthy lives.

Mary's advocacy has also played a significant role in advancing diabetes research and treatment. Her work has contributed to increased funding for diabetes research and the development of new therapies and technologies that have improved the lives of people with diabetes.

Though Mary has accomplished so much, she is the first to acknowledge that there is still much more work to be done. She remains committed to her mission of improving diabetes education and access to care, and encourage others to join in the fight against diabetes.

Mary's story is a reminder that with perseverance, education, and advocacy, individuals with chronic conditions can not only manage their conditions but thrive, and make a positive impact on the world.

Mary's work has had a ripple effect, inspiring others to become advocates for diabetes education and access to care. Her legacy will continue to inspire future generations to work towards a world free from the burden of diabetes.

Through her efforts, Mary has shown that even in the face of adversity, it is possible to create meaningful change and impact lives for the better. Her story is a reminder that every individual has the power to make a difference, and that together, we can work towards a brighter, healthier future.

Mary's work has also highlighted the importance of community and support in managing chronic conditions. She has created a network of individuals who share their experiences, offer encouragement, and provide a sense of belonging to those affected by diabetes.

This sense of community has not only improved mental health and well-being of those living with diabetes but has also fostered a sense of responsibility and accountability among individuals, reinforcing the importance of self-care and proactive management.

Mary's advocacy for diabetes education and access to care has undoubtedly had a significant impact on the lives of millions of people worldwide. Her legacy serves as an inspiration for others to continue the fight against diabetes and to work towards creating a world where individuals affected by chronic conditions can thrive.

In addition, Mary's work has brought attention to the need for more research into diabetes prevention and treatment, as well as the importance of addressing health disparities and improving access to healthcare.

Her advocacy has also inspired policy changes and initiatives aimed at improving diabetes care, such as increased funding for diabetes research and education programs, and the development of new diabetes treatments and technologies.

Mary's legacy is one of determination, passion, and compassion. Her tireless efforts to improve the lives of individuals with diabetes are a testament to the power of activism and advocacy. Her impact will continue to be felt for generations to come, as her work inspires others to make a difference and strive towards a future where everyone has the support and resources they need to thrive.

Mary has also been a strong voice in advocating for diabetes awareness globally. Her efforts have helped to increase public knowledge of the disease, including its causes, symptoms, and treatment options.

Through her work, Mary has also emphasized the importance of early detection and prevention of diabetes. She has encouraged regular check-ups, healthy lifestyle choices, and education at risk factors.

One of Mary's greatest contributions has been her ability to bring together individuals and organizations from diverse backgrounds to collaborate on diabetes initiatives. She has created partnerships between healthcare professionals, researchers, advocacy groups, and private sectors, all working towards a common goal of improving diabetes care and outcomes.

Mary's legacy serves as an inspiration to all those affected by diabetes, as well as to future generations of advocates and activists. Her vision of a world where diabetes is prevented, managed, and ultimately cured will continue to fuel the fight against this chronic disease for many years to come.

Mary has also been vocal about the importance of mental health in the diabetes community. She has highlighted the emotional toll of living with a chronic illness and has called for increased support and resources for those struggling with mental health issues related to their diabetes.

Additionally, Mary has been a champion of diversity and inclusion within the diabetes community. She has advocated for representation of all races, genders, and socioeconomic backgrounds in diabetes research, education, and care.

Through her leadership and tireless advocacy, Mary has become a recognized and respected figure in the diabetes community. Her contributions have made a significant impact on the lives of countless individuals affected by diabetes and her legacy will continue to inspire and propel the fight against this chronic disease.

Mary's work in promoting mental health awareness in the context of diabetes has been especially crucial, as living with this disease can take a toll on a person's emotional well-being. She has highlighted the need for support systems, therapy and counseling services, and other resources to help individuals manage the psychological effects of diabetes.

Moreover, Mary has stressed the importance of understanding the unique experiences of individuals from diverse backgrounds when it comes to diabetes care. She has emphasized the need for culturally competent care, as well as for involving people with diabetes in decision-making processes.

Mary's commitment to these important issues has helped to create a more inclusive and supportive diabetes community. Her legacy as an advocate for diabetes awareness and education will undoubtedly continue to inspire change and progress in the years to come.

Mary's leadership and advocacy have been instrumental in driving improvements in diabetes care, education, and research. Her dedication to mental health awareness and diversity and inclusion has helped to empower patients and foster a greater sense of community within the diabetes community.

Mary's voice will continue to be an important one in diabetes advocacy, and her example serves as an inspiration for others to follow. Her tireless work to raise awareness, educate, and support individuals with diabetes and their families will undoubtedly continue to make a difference in the fight against this chronic disease.

Short Success Story 22: A Woman

One short success story about diabetes is the case of a woman who was diagnosed with type 2 diabetes and was able to manage her condition with lifestyle changes. She made small changes like reducing the amount of sugar she consumed, increasing her physical activity, and losing weight. Over time, she was able to lower her blood sugar levels to a healthy range and was able to reduce the amount of medication she was taking for diabetes. She continued to follow a healthy lifestyle and was able to maintain her blood sugar levels without medication. This success story shows that with effort and dedication, it is possible to manage and even reverse type 2 diabetes through lifestyle changes.

Short Success Story 23: A Man

Another short success story is about a man in his early 50s who was diagnosed with diabetes. Instead of relying on medications alone, he decided to make significant changes to his diet and lifestyle. He switched to a plant-based diet and started exercising regularly. He also incorporated stress-reducing techniques like meditation and yoga into his daily routine. Within a few months, his blood sugar levels had significantly improved, and he was able to reduce his medication dosage. Over time, he was eventually able to stop taking medication altogether and managed his diabetes purely through diet and lifestyle changes. His success story proves that diabetes can be managed with a holistic approach that includes diet, exercise, and stress management.

Short Success Story 24: A Teenager

Another short success story is about a teenager who was diagnosed with type 1 diabetes. Despite the initial shock, she decided to take control of her condition and started learning everything she could about diabetes management. She worked closely with her healthcare provider to develop an individualized plan that incorporated insulin therapy, healthy eating, and regular exercise. She also joined a support group for people with diabetes and found a community of people who understood her struggles. With hard work and dedication, she was able to manage her blood glucose levels effectively and completed high school with honors. Her success story shows that with the right mindset, education, and support, people with diabetes can lead fulfilling and successful lives.

Short Success Story 25: A Young Girl

One short success story is about a young girl who was diagnosed with type 1 diabetes at the age of six. With the help of her parents and healthcare team, she quickly learned how to manage her condition and incorporated healthy habits into her everyday routine. She learned how to count carbs and adjust her insulin doses, as well as the importance of keeping active and eating a balanced diet. Despite the challenges of living with diabetes, she remained optimistic and never let her condition hold her back. She became an advocate for diabetes awareness and even started a fundraiser to support diabetes research. Today, she is a happy and healthy teenager with diabetes who is thriving both academically and socially. Her success story shows that even children can learn to manage diabetes with the right support and guidance.

Short Success Story 26: Another Man

One success story is about a man who was diagnosed with type 2 diabetes and struggled to manage his condition for years. He had trouble sticking to a healthy diet and exercise routine, which led to his blood sugar levels fluctuating and causing him to feel unwell. However, after attending a diabetes management program, he began to make small but meaningful changes to his lifestyle. He started by incorporating more fruits and vegetables into his diet and going for short walks after meals to help regulate his blood sugar levels. Over time, he began to notice significant improvements in his health and started to feel better than ever before. He also began to inspire others in his community to manage their diabetes and make positive changes to their lifestyles. Today, he is in control of his diabetes and is living a fulfilling life with a renewed sense of hope and purpose.

He also began to attend support groups for people with diabetes, where he could share his experiences with others who understood what he was going through. Through these groups, he learned about new treatment options and strategies for managing his condition. He also made new friends and found a sense of community, which helped him stay motivated and committed to his health.

As he continued to make progress, he decided to set new health and wellness goals for himself, such as running a 5K race and learning how to cook healthy meals. He started to measure his success by the positive changes he was making in his life, rather than just his blood sugar levels or other medical markers.

Through his journey with diabetes, this man learned that managing a chronic condition requires a holistic approach that addresses both physical and emotional health. He learned to take small steps every day towards better health, and to celebrate his successes along the way. And he is grateful every day for the support, encouragement and inspiration he found in others with diabetes; there is a whole community of people who know how to turn adversity into strength, and he is proud to be a part of it.

In addition to the support he found in his diabetes community, this man also discovered the importance of a supportive family. He talked openly with his wife and children about his diabetes, and they too rose to the challenge of making healthy choices and supporting his goals. His wife even started participating in 5K races with him!

Together, this man and his family have made healthy living a priority in their lives. They experiment with new recipes, go on daily walks, and find fun ways to stay active as a family. And while living with diabetes is still a daily challenge, this man feels confident that he has the tools, knowledge, and support he needs to live a happy, healthy life. He knows that with the right support and mindset, anyone can overcome obstacles and achieve their wellness goals.

As he reflects on his journey with diabetes, this man is grateful for the lessons he has learned through his experiences. He has learned the power of the community, both in terms of finding support and sharing his own experiences with others. He has also learned the importance of taking a holistic approach to health, focusing not just on medical markers but on small, everyday choices that add up over time.

Most importantly, though, this man has learned that living with a chronic condition does not have to define him. With the right mindset, he can lead a full and active life, pursuing his passions and achieving his goals. And he hopes that by sharing his story, he can inspire others to do the same.

He wants people to know that they are not alone in their struggles, and that seeking support and education can make a significant difference in their health outcomes and quality of life. He encourages everyone to take their health seriously and make small changes necessary to live a healthy and fulfilling life.

In the end, this man is proof that with the right attitude, mindset, and support system, anyone can overcome obstacles and achieve their wellness goals. He is proud of how far he has come in his journey with diabetes, and he knows that he has the strength and determination to face any challenges that come his way.

He also recognizes that diabetes and other chronic conditions require ongoing management and that it is essential to continue to prioritize health and wellness every day. He plans to continue working with his healthcare team and using the resources available to him to stay on top of his condition and maintain optimal health.

Overall, this man's story is one of resilience, hope, and perseverance. He hopes that it can serve as a source of inspiration and encouragement for anyone else struggling with a chronic health condition. With the right mindset and support, anyone can overcome the challenges of living with a chronic illness and lead a fulfilling and meaningful life.

He also recognizes that diabetes and other chronic conditions require ongoing management and that it is essential to continue to prioritize health and wellness every day. He plans to continue working with his healthcare team and using the resources available to him to stay on top of his condition and maintain optimal health.

Overall, this man's story is one of resilience, hope, and perseverance. He hopes that it can serve as a source of inspiration and encouragement for anyone else struggling with a chronic health condition. With the right mindset and support, anyone can overcome the challenges of living with a chronic illness and lead a fulfilling and meaningful life.

The key to success in managing diabetes is consistent self-care and working closely with healthcare professionals to create and follow a personal care plan. This includes regularly monitoring blood sugar levels, taking medication as prescribed, following a healthy diet and exercise routine, and avoiding unhealthy habits like smoking and excessive alcohol consumption. It's also crucial to educate oneself about diabetes and how it affects the body, along with learning how to manage symptoms and prevent complications. Developing a support system of family and friends who encourage and motivate a person can also contribute to long-term success in managing diabetes. Ultimately, the most important factor is a commitment to self-care and making healthy choices every day, which can help individuals with diabetes live full and active lives.

The key failure of diabetes management can be attributed to several factors, including poor control over blood sugar levels, lack of knowledge about the disease and its management, failure to make necessary lifestyle changes, and inadequate medical treatment.

One of the main causes of diabetes management failure is poor control over blood sugar levels. This can occur due to a variety of reasons, such as unhealthy eating habits, lack of exercise, medication non-adherence, or insulin resistance. As a result, diabetic patients may experience high or low blood sugar levels which can lead to serious health complications if left unchecked.

Another significant factor that contributes to diabetes management failure is a lack of knowledge. Many diabetic patients are not aware of the various aspects of diabetes management and how to effectively manage their symptoms. They may not understand how to monitor their blood sugar levels or what foods to eat and avoid. Without proper education, it can be difficult to achieve and maintain good control over blood sugar levels.

Furthermore, failure to make necessary lifestyle changes can also lead to poor diabetes management. This includes making dietary changes, engaging in regular physical activity, quitting smoking, and managing stress. Without these lifestyle modifications, it can be difficult to achieve long-term blood sugar control.

Lastly, inadequate medical treatment and monitoring can also contribute to diabetes management failure. Diabetic patients should have regular appointments with their healthcare providers to monitor their blood sugar levels, adjust medications, and identify any potential complications early on. Failure to access such regular care can impede effective diabetes management.

Conclusion

In conclusion, the short success stories in this book prove that with the right mindset, support, and management strategies, living with diabetes can lead to a fulfilling and rewarding life. The individuals featured in these stories have faced challenges and obstacles, but through perseverance, education, and self-care, they have thrived and achieved their goals.

The stories also serve as a source of hope and inspiration to anyone navigating life with diabetes. With proper management, a positive attitude, and the support of family, friends, and healthcare professionals, life with diabetes can be a journey of success and fulfillment. We hope that the stories in this book have encouraged and empowered you to make positive changes in your own life and to continue to strive for success in your diabetes management.

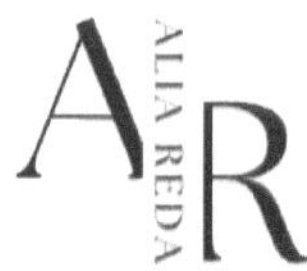